I0412030

Breast Cancer Wellness

The Breast Cancer Survival Guide

By: Rabhu Gudapati MD

[978-1511754194]

TABLE OF CONTENTS

PUBLISHERS NOTES

Disclaimer

This publication is intended to provide helpful and informative material. It is not intended to diagnose, treat, cure, or prevent any health problem or condition, nor is intended to replace the advice of a physician. No action should be taken solely on the contents of this book. Always consult your physician or qualified healthcare professional on any matters regarding your health and before adopting any suggestions in this book or drawing inferences from it.

The author and publisher specifically disclaim all responsibility for any liability, loss or risk, personal or otherwise, which is incurred as a consequence, directly or indirectly, from the use or application of any contents of this book.

Any product names referenced within this book are the trademarks of their respective owners. None of these owners have sponsored, authorized, endorsed, or approved this book.

Always read all information provided by the manufacturers' product labels before using their products. The author and publisher are not responsible for claims made by manufacturers.

Paperback Edition

Manufactured in the United States of America

CHAPTER 1- CHAPTER 1 WHAT IS BREAST CANCER?

Breast cancer is a serious health condition in which cancer cells grow and spread throughout the breast tissue. The breast is made up of millions of cells. At any point during your life, those cells are rotating between resting period and growth periods. This growth is actually controlled by the very center of each cell. This center is called the cell's nucleus. Specifically, the nucleus has genes located within it that control the way the cells develop. When it is working in good condition, the cells are healthy and functioning as they should. But, when there are abnormalities in the way the cells grow and develop, there is little control over the periods of rest and growth in the cell. Whenever there is uncontrolled growth in these cells, breast cancer forms.

Breast cancer is not just a condition for women, either. Breast cancer in men is possible. Cancer is sometimes caused by hereditary. Many times, this is not the case, though. In fact, according to some studies, up to 90 percent of all breast cancer cases are caused by the natural aging process as well as the lifestyle that you are living. This makes it important for every woman to consider if they could become a victim of this disease. Learning the breast cancer statistics can help you see just how prevalent the condition is. In addition, you should know your family's history. If you have had a mother or grandmother or even an aunt that has had breast cancer, you are more likely to get it as well.

Learning as much as you can about breast cancer is important. Breast cancer facts are readily available, too. As research happens and changes, you are sure to see that there are opportunities for you to learn even more. Staying up to date on breast cancer can be a challenge, for anyone, simply because there are so many new things happening. A good place to be, though, is at your doctor's office yearly for a checkup. Also, ask your doctor to show you how to check for breast cancer on your own. Through simply tests each month, you can help assure yourself of not becoming another one of the cancer fatalities.

One of the most important things to know about breast cancer is the signs of breast cancer. If you are struggling with this condition, you know fully what the risks are. Yet, for those that may not have experienced it before, know the signs and get yourself to a doctor as soon as you believe you could be at risk. Early detection of breast cancer is the best way to fight it and to overcome it.

What is breast cancer? It is a type of disease that grows inside of you, due to the abnormal growth of cells in your body. These cancer cells can be highly detrimental to your overall health, and worse, they can easily spread to other portions of your body. This is why it is so important to have all the breast cancer information out there and to make good decisions about your health.

CHAPTER 2- FACTS OF BREAST CANCER: WHAT DOCTORS ARE DOING?

Do you have all the breast cancer facts you need? If you are a women, then you need to consider breast cancer a serious threat to your life, even if you do not have any women in your family that have had it.

Breast cancer is not something that has to be passed down from one generation to the next. While it can be, there are various other causes of breast cancer that are just as worrisome. Knowing a few facts about breast cancer can help you to overcome the situation and improve your chances of survival.

Who Can Get It?

Breast cancer awareness is one of the most important aspects of the condition. Many women do realize that they can suffer from breast cancer. Yet, they can. Every month, you should do a self exam of yourself, at the same day of your cycle as the previous month. This will allow you to notice any lumps in the breast tissue that are not normal. For most people, there are going to be some normal lumps in the tissue, but these are not cancerous. What you need to be concerned with is the lumps that have not been there in the past. Besides this, you also need to consider the likelihood of having some type of breast cancer screening done every year by your doctor.

Anyone can get breast cancer. In fact, this condition is not just one that women face. Men can also suffer from breast cancer, though it is much rarer. In many cases, doctors do not know what causes the breast cancer to happen, either.

Signs To Monitor For

As you do your self-exam each month, you'll notice any changes in the breast tissue. Since the breasts change throughout your menstrual cycle, these can be hard to detect unless you do the test every day on the same day of the month. In addition to this, you need to look at your breast tissue in general. Many people have swollen or painful skin here which could be a sign of a problem, especially if there are no other reasons for the irritation. Additionally, if you have any type of pain in your breast or this region of the body, talk to your doctor about it. Know the signs of breast cancer.

Treatment Is Out There

Another misconception about breast cancer is that there are not many treatments available to those that have this condition. Some people believe that they will lose their breasts if they have the disease in surgery. While this can happen, most people do not have it happen to them. Having the correct breast cancer information is important. Doctors have a full arsenal of helpful treatment options available to them to help overcome this disease. There are drugs used, hormonal treatments, radiation, complimentary medications as well as chemotherapy, all of which can be very beneficial in the treatment of breast cancer. Even for those with stage 4 breast cancer, there is help available to them.

Perhaps the most important breast cancer facts to let other women know include the fact that you need to be monitored and checked regularly for this condition. Early detection of the breast cancer is the best way to overcome it. Time and time again, doctors are able to treat patients that have these early stages because they have done the self checkups and have found the lumps. Get in to see your doctor yearly and have a professional checkup done that will examine any of the risk factors you have for developing breast cancer. With your doctor's help, you'll be able to fight off this disease.

Causes: Still Unknown

Doctors do not know the causes of breast cancer in most cases. Doctors do know that many women will experience breast cancer, with the number of cases every year rising. Yet, researchers are working to learn more about this disease including what they can do to overcome it. Many times, doctors are able to improve the condition simply by using the various treatments available. Success rates for treatment drugs and methods are improving. Yet, doctors are consistently looking for ways to improve the overall well being of patients suffering this condition. To do that, they need to know the causes of it.

What Risks Are There?

While doctors do not always understand the cause of breast cancer, they do have a good ideal of the risks of breast cancer. They know that there are various types of conditions and situations in which breast cancer symptoms develop. Here is a closer look at some of these.

Gender: Both men and women can get breast cancer, though men are much less likely. While about 200,000 cases of breast cancer in women are seen each year, only about 2000 or less are reported in men. If you are a woman, you need to realize the risks are here.

Age: The older you are, the more risk you have for developing breast cancer. Studies show that two out of three women that have invasive breast cancer have gotten it at the age of 55 or more. This is believed to be caused by the breast tissues simply wearing down over time.

Genetics: Some of the latest research shows that genes do play a role in getting cancer in the breast. Doctors have been able to pinpoint various genes that play a role in this development. In fact, those genes are BRCA1 and BRCA2. When there are mutations in these genes, cancer may form.

Hereditary: If you do have a family history of breast cancer, your chances of getting breast cancer are higher than those that do not. Yet, this is not the only reason for getting cancer and only a small portion of those cases reported are actually those women who have relatives with it as well.

Past breast cancer: If you have had breast cancer in the past, you are more likely to have another case than those women that have not had it at all.

Race: Women of all races are able to get breast cancer, but those that are white have a slightly increased chance of having breast cancer than African American women. But, African American women with breast cancer are more likely to die from the cancer, because research shows these tumors seem to grow faster in these people. Others, including Asians, American Indians and Hispanic women have less of a chance of getting breast cancer.

Why is it important for doctors to know these risk factors? Knowing the symptoms of breast cancer can save your life. In fact, doctors are able to get help to those that need it the most by weighing these risk factors and helping those patients with them to be screened for breast cancer more often. Early detection is the single most important tool in the fight against the disease, and doctors are able to help patients when they know what these signs are.

If you are suffering from breast cancer, or believe you could be, talk to your doctor. Those that have these risks of breast cancer, or know they have some of the causes of breast cancer in their lives, should get help as soon as possible.

CHAPTER 3- STATISTICS: WHAT'S HAPPENING IN THIS FIELD?

Breast cancer statistics show that there is an increasing number of people suffering from breast cancer each year. Yet, through a good understanding of this disease a well as the treatment options available for it getting larger, more of these cancers are treated and overcome by patients. If you have been diagnosed with cancer, you still can overcome this health risk, even if you have later stages of the condition. Choosing the best treatment option for you is the best route to take, and your doctor will help make that happen.

Latest Research

Doctors are continuously working on breast cancer research. They are developing new methods for treating this condition constantly, and they are likely making some good breakthroughs. One area they are working on improving is the overall success rate of medications in the breast cancer stages. For example, in stage iv breast cancer, some treatment options may no longer work. Yet, doctors are working on new treatments that can be effective.

If you are suffering from breast cancer, and are interested, you may be able to learn more about these research opportunities. You may be able to help by being a part of the study and learning more about the condition in general. Doctors often find that patients who participate in research studies are more confident in overcoming their condition, and they are not usually put at risk. Talk to your doctor about any studies happening in the hospital or medical area in your area.

How Many People?

The latest breast cancer statistics show that an estimated 250,000 cases of breast cancer are identified each year, and that number is growing. In addition to this, there also are more cases of breast cancer in men. While this condition is still very rare, with only about 2000 cases a year being diagnosed, men need to be aware that it can happen to them. Treatment options are available for men that are suffering from this type of cancer, too, and they are highly likely to be effective.

The number of people that have breast cancer may be growing in part by the measures of the breast cancer awareness teams that are helping more women learn how to do breast self exams. These exams are one of the best ways to detect breast cancer in patients, and they are one of the best ways to catch it early. Doctors say that those who are suffering from breast cancer have a better chance at survival if they are, in fact, able to be treated in the early stages of cancer. These self exams can help people catch their cancer at this stage.

Treatments Flourish

Another important piece of information about breast cancer is that the number of treatment options available to doctors is increasing. Patients can get complimentary treatments as well. These treatments include methods that work with your current doctor prescribed treatments. For example, some have seen success with acupuncture, yoga as well as meditation.

While those treatments are helpful, the number of other treatments involving medical signs is even more. Doctor can now treat breast cancer with medications and drugs of varying sorts, with hormonal treatments, with radiation and much more.

There is no doubt that having the right treatment is the most important thing for doctors in lowering the mortality rate in patients with breast cancer. Breast cancer statistics show that more people are overcoming this condition every year, and that with continued support and research, doctors will be able to continue finding new ways to treat this condition. For those who are suffering from breast cancer, these are important words to hear.

CHAPTER 4- SIGNS AND SYMPTOMS OF BREAST CANCER

Do you know what the signs and symptoms of breast cancer are? If not, and you are a women, you could be putting your life on the line. Many people mistakenly believe cancer will not happen to them, and often this is the biggest mistake to make. You do not have to have a family member that has suffered through this disease to go through it yourself. You do not have to have a bad lifestyle, smoke or even work in a factory to get this type of cancer. In fact, it targets millions of people every year without any warning at all. Knowing the breast cancer symptoms can save your life.

Sometimes breast cancer is very hard to detect. Not all cancers will actually have symptoms that present themselves to you. The best way to know if these cancers are present then is through testing. As you age, you are more likely to develop breast cancer, which means that you should be tested for breast cancer often once you are at menopause and beyond. Doctors recommended the first screenings for breast cancer to happen at the age of 35 to 40, depending on your age.

Before this time, you should still have doctor examinations that could point out any lumps in the tissue or other worrisome conditions. Once you reach an older age, you'll need doctors to do full screenings on you, including tests like mammograms, which will take pictures of your breast and pinpoint any problems that may exist. Even if you have no breast cancer symptoms, you still need to have these tests done after you reach this age to help you improve your chances of detection.

Sometimes, there are breast cancer signs. These signs will range widely based on the type of situation you are in as well as the overall size of the cancer in your body. Some symptoms of breast cancer include:

- Lumps in the breasts that are not normal, or are present throughout the month (your breast may have some small lumps in it at some times during the month because of your menstrual cycle).
- The skin around your breast and on your breast may swell and show the signs of inflammation as well as the lumps themselves.
- Pain in the breast area which may be the result of the lump an inflammation.

If you feel that you may be experiencing any of these symptoms, you'll need to talk to your doctor about it as soon as possible. Doctors will perform a number of tests to make a diagnosis. It is not always easy to make these decisions from first exams, which is very frustrating for many women. Nevertheless, you'll need to have the right information when it comes to breast cancer.

When a diagnosis is made and you have been told you have breast cancer, you and your doctors will determine the best treatments for breast cancer. This process can sometimes take some time as well. Yet, through treatment you can beat the cancer and get on with your life.

Talk to your doctor about any signs and symptoms of breast cancer that you may have. The sooner you talk to them about the condition, the sooner you can get help for it. Best of all, most cases of potential breast cancer are not going to actually be it. Periodically check yourself each month and you'll be well on your way to protecting yourself from the onset of cancer. Doctors will be happy to show you the proper way to give yourself these check ups.

CHAPTER 5- WHAT WILL HAPPEN DURING TREATMENT?

Breast cancer treatment will be tailored to your specific situation. Doctors first must determine if you have the cancer, how much you have and how fast it is spreading. There are also various types of cancer you could be suffering from. The effectiveness of any treatment is determined in part by your condition, but many of these treatments are highly effective. Here is an overview of the types of treatment available to you, though there are many sub levels of treatment available as well.

Local and Regional Treatment

A local treatment or a regional treatment is one of the most specific types of treatment available. Here, the actual location of the cancer is targeted directly. This can be done through various drugs, but may also include surgery for breast cancer. Regional treatments are those that refer to treatments of the lymph nodes as well as the breast tissue. If your condition metastasis, which means that it has spread to other areas of the body, then it becomes important for this treatment option to include those regions as well. Common locations of spreading include he lungs or even your bones.

Systemic Treatments

Sometimes, treatments must be used that target the entire body. These are Systemic treatments. The most common treatment for breast cancer that falls under this area is chemotherapy. Chemotherapy is an example of this type of treatment. Breast cancer chemotherapy works by injecting drugs into the body that will fight off the cancer cells. Breast cancer drug use is common because it can be highly effective. Most of the time, chemotherapy is made up of a variety of types of breast cancer drugs, but one can be used solely as well. Doctors determine which drugs to use based on the overall situation in your body.

How Chemotherapy Helps

Chemotherapy is like a cocktail filled with various types of drugs. Since all of your body's cells are growing at different times, this type of treatment can target just those cells growing at a specific point. Cancer cells area always growing and changing, which means they will be attacked by this type of drug treatment. Any and all cells that are actively growing in your body will likely die during the chemotherapy treatment. This really does exhaust the body and it can be one of the most painful situations you experience because of the intensity. Yet, it is also highly effective at removing any growing cancer cells in your body.

What's Going To Work?

One of the most difficult aspects of getting help for breast cancer is that sometimes the treatment for breast cancer does not work for everyone. The advanced stages of the cancer can sometimes cause a number of problems in and of itself. More so, the body will react differently to medications in some situations. Every person must be thoroughly evaluated and, unfortunately, there is no way to know which type of treatment will work best for your type of cancer until doctors rely on their experience and their ability to test various drugs.

Advances in medicine are always happening. In fact, more doctors than ever are able to get the help they need in fighting breast cancer by using new methods of medication and treatment. As you talk to your doctor and analyze the treatment options for your needs, ask about alternative treatments, experimental treatments and other options available to you. Being aggressive in treating breast cancer is the best way to fight it and keeping a positive mind set and goals is also the best way to make that treatment successful. The right breast cancer treatment for you is out there, you just need to find it.

Understand What's Happening during Chemotherapy

Breast cancer chemotherapy is a treatment option for those suffering from breast cancer. In this treatment, a variety of drugs for cancer are used. The goal is to kill off the cancer cells in the body to keep the disease from spreading and actually to cure it from the body's tissues. Chemotherapy is called a systemic treatment because it is used to treat the entire body from cancer, and the drugs used during the process will affect cells throughout your body. The good news is that chemotherapy is one of the most effective types of treatments that doctors have in improving your chances of getting through this disease.

How It Works?

If you will have chemotherapy treatment, your doctor will talk to you about how the process works, and will tell you what the specific drugs used in the treatment will be. Generally, the medications chosen to be part of the chemotherapy treatment are based on the type and amount of cancer you have, and the medications that are available to treat it. The term chemotherapy is a term used to describe the drugs used to treat your cancer, but it can be one drug or several drugs working together. One thing is sure about any chemotherapy treatment and that is that it is highly toxic to the body. The goal of this treatment is to kill cancer cells, which will cause the rest of your body to also be affected.

When you have cancer of any type, your body has cells that do not grow correctly. Cancer cells grow very quickly and split often. This growing and splitting is not normal because normal healthy cells have periods of rest. Yet, as these cells grow and split over and over again, they produce the tumors and lumps you may feel. The job of chemotherapy drugs is to wipe out any cells in your body that are working on splitting. These drugs are selected for their ability to target only those cells in your body that are dividing.

There are other cells in your body that are also dividing, which may cause them to become targets as well. For example, the cells found in your mouth, in your blood, in your hair, vagina, and nails are healthy cells that divide often as well. For this reason, chemotherapy patients often experience painful sores or problems with these areas of the body due to their chemotherapy treatment. For example, many women will lose their hair because of the chemotherapy for breast cancer. Yet, that doesn't mean that your hair always falls out, as some medications do not cause this. What does happen in these treatments is that the cancer is killed off.

There are various types of breast cancer, many of which can be treated with chemotherapy. Doctors will tailor the medications you take by the types of cancers you have as well as the size and location of it. When it comes to a breast cancer treatment, chemotherapy is often used, but it is not always an option for patients. In some situations, the right breast cancer treatments may include removing the tumor from your body or using other methods. Doctors will need to determine the right treatment for you, specifically.

For those suffering from breast cancer, chemotherapy treatment is one of the best tools doctors have to help you overcome it. Yet, it will do damage to your body. Many times, these drugs are highly effective while other times they are likely to cause you to feel warn out and tired. Over time, these side effects will improve.

CHAPTER 6- THE IMPORTANCE OF AWARENESS FOR BREAST CANCER

Breast cancer awareness is one of the most important things for women of all ages, races and situations to know about. This type of cancer is troublesome because it often is not detected until there is a sizable lump in the breast tissue, which can signify the onset of the condition. Anyone that is concerned with their health in terms of if this condition could be affecting them should seek medical treatment as soon as possible. If you are unsure of what breast cancer is, you should take some time to learn more about it.

What Is Breast Cancer?

Unbelievably, many people do not know what breast cancer is. It is often thought of as a silent killer because there are very few symptoms of breast cancer. Many times, it can go undetected for months before you notice that something is not right and get to a doctor. Cancer is a type of disease in which the cells in the body do not develop correctly. Unlike normal cells, the genes of cancer cells continuously tell them to grow and develop, whereas with normal, healthy cells, there are periods of growth and periods of non growth. Because the cancer cells continue to grow, the develop clusters which can invade the surrounding tissue and even spread to other areas of the body. Over time, they can threaten major organs and become lethal.

Getting Breast Cancer Aware

If you do not know much about breast cancer, you are not alone. Millions of people each year first learn of this disease when their doctors tell them they have it. What's important to note is that the disease can and will spread if it is not taken care of as soon as possible. Early detection of cancer is the best way to overcome the condition, too.

You can get breast cancer information from several locations. First, make an appointment with your family doctor or your gynecologist. They will perform a check up on your to examine any potential problems you could be facing. During this test, doctors will also show you how to perform a self diagnostic test. This test should be done very month on the same day of your cycle. If you feel anything that is not appropriate or that could be a lump, you should call your doctor right away to get a full check up.

There are many doctors working on breast cancer research on any given day. Their goal is to find better methods to curing the disease. The causes of breast cancer are another area they are working hard on. Unfortunately, it is not always understood why some people experience breast cancer and others do not. Yet, it is always a highly worrisome situation when you do. As doctors look for better medications to treat breast cancer, you can rest assured that you'll be protected if and when these new medications become known. Yet, in the meantime, you have to be a self monitor for yourself and those women you know who are at a potential risk.

There are many reasons to be concerned about breast cancer. The statistics of breast cancer show that there are many millions of Americans suffering from this disease every year and millions more throughout the world. While doctors race to find ways to improve the condition, it becomes just as important for people to be proactive in their treatment and in their breast cancer awareness. If you are passionate, help raise funds to support breast cancer research. You may find yourself in need of this help and the new knowledge doctors have one day.

CHAPTER 7- SURGERY FOR BREAST CANCER: WHAT, WHY, AND HOW

Breast cancer surgery is often considered one of the first methods of treating breast cancer. Doctors are able to help patients in this way by removing the breast cancer cells growing in the region, therefore, removing the problem altogether. The way that surgery for breast cancer is done has change, though. Over the last ten years, doctors have refined their methods and made the surgery much more refined and to the point. In doing so, they have been able to improve the overall health and well being of the individual, while still improving the overall look of the breast.

Will You Have It?

Surgery is often considered one of the best breast cancer treatment options. In this type of cancer, the cancer cells continue to grow and split rapidly, which often forms a tumor. As the tumor grows and the cancer spreads, it can destroy the health and well being of your organs and skin. By removing the tumor and infected breast tissue through surgery, doctors can effectively stop the process and start improving your life. Generally, surgery is used in one of two forms:

Breast Conserving Surgery: In this type of surgery, doctors target only a small portion of the breast where the breast cancer has been found. They remove just the tumor or the lump (called a lumpectomy) and the rest of the breast is left in place. For those that have a small, localized area of exposure, this is the best method of treatment available.

Mastectomy: Another type of breast surgery is a mastectomy when much of the breast it removed. This is often a more drastic measure, but in most cases, doctors will only use it as a last result. For cancers located in various portions of the breast, this may be a necessary, life saving procedure.

Coupling Treatments

In most situations, there will be a combined effort to fight off the breast cancer. Doctors will need to work through various treatments even if surgery is used to remove the breast tissue. When they do this, they are effectively killing as many of the cancer cells as possible, giving you the best chance at survival.

If you have a breast surgery to remove a tumor or even the entire breast, you will likely have radiation along with it. The radiation can be targeted to the region of the body. When the doctors include both of these methods, he has increased your ability to survive, since radiation will destroy all the remaining tissues in the region which are cancerous.

In addition to this, sometimes it is necessary for doctors to consider chemotherapy for breast cancer. This type of breast cancer drugs mix is used to help target the remaining cancer cells. Chemotherapy treatments are used because these drugs are able to kill and destroy any cells in the body which are growing and splitting. While this may cause side effects including hair loss, it also helps to stop the cancer cells, as these cancer cells are known for their ability to reproduce very quickly. When doctors combine these treatments, they are looking for the most aggressive methods to overcoming the condition. In many cases, they work very well.

If you are likely to have breast cancer surgery, ask your doctor about your options. Full mastectomies are not as common as they used to be, as doctors are able to save much of the breast tissue that has not become infected. Yet, doctors will need to treat you for the type and level of breast cancer you have, which may require a specialized treatment. Talk to your doctor about your options.

CHAPTER 8- TREATMENTS USED IN BREAST CANCER TREATMENT

With breast cancer drug options available, doctors can and do treat breast cancer effectively. There are various types of drugs and other treatment options available to doctors and everyone can benefit from them. If you are suffering from breast cancer, chances are good your doctor has determined the best medications to help with your case. The selection of these medications is based on the type of breast cancer you have as well as the overall stage and level of health that you have. Many factors play a role in which type of treatment is used, but most of them are highly effective.

Treatment Options Available

Doctors have a wide range of drug treatments that can be effective. Even in situations of metastatic breast cancer, you will find options to consider. Here is a look at some of the treatments for breast cancer available.

- **Surgery:** In some cases, surgery for breast tissue removal is the best option for your situation. By removing the infected breast tissues, doctors can remove the tumors that are present as well as any other tissue that could become infected. This is one of the best options for overcoming the condition.
- **Radiation therapy:** Doctors may choose to use radiation to kill the growing breast cancer cells. There are various advantages of this condition and it is often a very successful treatment, even though it has some of the worst side effects.
- **Hormonal treatment:** Doctors have been able to use hormones to treat the breast cancer. There are a number of different types

available to them including ERD's, SERM's and aromatase inhibitors. These have been shown to be highly effective.

- **Breast cancer chemotherapy:** Doctors know that treating breast cancer with a variety of different breast cancer drugs can be highly effective. These treatments will kill any splitting cells in the body, of which cancer cells are. While the side effects can be harsh, it is usually an effective treatment.
- **Complimentary treatments:** Your doctor may or may not consider these, but you can. Treatments like meditation, yoga and even acupuncture are helpful in allowing the body to heal. Don't stop your current drug treatment program or the methods your doctor is using to use these treatments, but couple your current treatment with these complimentary ones.

When doctors find that you have breast cancer signs, they will need to consider further testing before they can determine if you need treatment and what type of treatment is best for you. The right breast cancer drug is available, more than likely, to help improve your situation. If you are unsure of the breast cancer facts of the medication your doctor is giving you, you can do some research on them individually. Drugs are used in various ways, and most often, they are used in combinations.

A good example of this combination of a variety of breast cancer drugs is in the treatment of chemotherapy. Doctors will select the most likely drugs that will work for your situation and administer them to you. In most treatments, these drugs work by killing any of the cancer cells or other cells in your body that are splitting.

Most people will be given at least one type of breast cancer drug to treat their condition, most will use several. Each drug has its own side effects and overall risks. Some are worse than others. Yet, losing your hair or having sores in your mouth can mean that the breast cancer in your body is being destroyed. This often is a worthwhile risk to take on. Talk to your doctor about the risks of the drug you are taking.

Keeping Updated about Research

Breast cancer research is a continuously fight that doctors, scientists and pharmacists are working hard one at all times. While breast cancer is a condition that doctors have medications to treat and many people are able to overcome it, the journey of detecting breast cancer and treating it more effectively has many opportunities for new treatments and better results. As doctors work to improve their knowledge of breast cancer, they will often do research studies and tests that you could become part of. Sometimes, the best medicine of all is to know that there are millions of people fighting for your successful recovery from this disease.

What They Are Working On

There are many things breast cancer research teams are working on. Here are some things you may be able to benefit from.

Early detection is known to be one of the best ways to overcome breast cancer. Doctors know that if they want to be successful at treating this condition that they'll need to provide you with the best methods for knowing the condition s there. To do this, doctors are working on new ways to effectively find a diagnosis breast cancer in women, and men, sooner. Some of the most amazing studies involve the use of DNA and determining if there is a link there.

Doctors are working on their ability to treat more advanced stages of breast cancer, such as stage 4 breast cancer. In later stages of the disease, there are fewer opportunities for doctors to treat the cancer with the medications that they have and many times chemotherapy is not as effective as it could be if it was done earlier. Many times, this is one of the worst situations for patients to find themselves in.

Doctors are working on learning new methods of treating breast cancer with surgery, too. Currently breast cancer surgery is a treatment option, but it is not always the best choice. Many times, doctors find that the cancer has spread to the rest of the body or that they cannot get to the cancer well enough. This can cause a number of problems for the patient, including the inability to fight off the condition. New breast cancer research is being done to improve surgery techniques including offering less invasive procedures.

Doctors are working on learning more about types of breast cancer that they do not know as much about. For example, they do not know as much as they ca about male breast cancer cases and why some men are affected by it. There are other types of cancers that doctors are trying to learn more about as well. The more they know about these treatments, the better they will be at treating this disease in patients.

The only way for doctors to do this type of research is through consistent methods of funding. Unfortunately, there is not always enough funds to make these changes happen. You can be part of helping people learn more about breast cancer by becoming an advocate for breast cancer. Help raise money and work on giving people the knowledge they need to get help for their condition.

Breast cancer research is ongoing, as there are still many things that doctors are working on learning more about. While there may be methods to getting cancer out of the body, the cure for all types of cancer are not here yet. As doctors get closer, though, you'll be able to see many more opportunities for advancements in the way doctors can fight this condition.

CHAPTER 9- TYPES OF BREAST CANCER

What Could Happen?

There are several types of breast cancer, defined by the stage they are in and the overall composition of them. If you are suffering from breast cancer, you should ask your doctor to tell you what type of cancer you have as well as what stage the cancer is in. There are treatment options available for most situations, depending on what stage of cancer you are in. Understanding these facts will help you get the most help for your health and improve your lifespan.

What Doctors Are Looking For

In a breast cancer diagnosis, doctors need to consider various factors about the actual cancer cells they find. The course of action they take to improve your health is based on these factors. Here are some things that they will look at.

What is the size of the cancer? Small lumps and tumors are often easier to treat and easier to overcome than others. Yet, if the tumor is larger, they will need to take more aggressive measures to treat it. A large tumor doesn't have to mean death, though.

What is the growth rate: Doctors will do breast cancer tests to help determine what the level of intensity of growth is. A fast growing, aggressive style of cancer needs more aggressive means of help. Some tumors are very low key and are easily treated, though.

What type of behavior does it have? In some situations, the behavior of a tumor can be predictable. In other words, doctors understand the way it is growing and the speed. Other situations are much more unpredictable, which can lead to other means of treatment.

Doctor will characterize the tumors of breast cancer by their size, the tumor grade, the hormone receptor status of the tumor, the margins of resection and the HER2/Neu oncogene overexpression. These elements may seem like a foreign language, but to doctors they can better tailor their treatment when they have as much information as possible.

There are other concerns with breast cancer as well. For example, male breast cancer is a type of cancer that forms in men. Men do have a limited amount of breast tissue, which can actually grow in size depending on the overall health and weight of an individual, their exposure to various outside elements as well as other factors. This type of cancer is rare, occurring in only 2000 or so cases per year.

In addition to this, doctors are also concerned about the metastatic breast cancer rates. Metastatic breast cancer is a type that spreads through the body by the blood stream. The cancer cells are able to break through the tissue and they can then spread to various areas of the body. When this happens, those cancer cells can latch onto various other organs n the body and in turn develop tumors in that region. This is a highly worrisome situation because the rate of additional complications is high.

Once doctors have a good understanding of the types of breast cancer they have to work with, they can choose the best treatment for breast cancer. Treatments are decided upon by the actual case, so what works for you may not be right for someone else. Doctors tailor your health to the cancer you have.

If you are suffering from breast cancer, ask your doctor more about what type of cancer you have. Learn as much as you can and consider alternative treatments that work in complimentary form to your current one. Doctors can help you overcome breast cancer with the help of these treatment options, most often being successful.

The Seriousness of Stage 4

Stage 4 breast cancer is one of the worst stages that you can have. In this stage, the cancer is very aggressive and has moved to be at its most dangerous form. Doctors will still provide you with excellent treatment options, and many patients do survive breast cancer at this stage. In this advanced form, though, there may be limits. Unfortunately, according to the American Cancer Society, there is only a 20 percent chance of survival beyond five years for people who have this stage of cancer.

What Are Stages

Doctors have developed a system of stages to help them know which level the breast cancer is in. In the earliest stages, the cancer is very small and often times go undetected. As the tumor grows in size, it will move up in terms of stage level. Stages range from stage 1 (or stage I) to stage 4 (or stage IV). There are also subdivisions in each stage. Doctors will rate the disease by size, but also by other factors including the amount and type of growth of the stage as well as the overall aggressiveness of the stage. Doctors are also concerned about the overall way that the tumor is growing. Most will grow in a "normal" pattern, which allows them to tailor treatment to that specific stage easier. Others are unpredictable and this often can be one of the most troublesome types of cancer.

Defining Stage

In order for doctors to know which breast cancer stage you are in, they will need to do a wide variety of tests. They will do this in the effort to fully understand the condition, so they can give you the best treatment options available. Generally, doctors will do tests that include x rays that are highly intense, as well as blood work and much more. Once they are confident that they know all there is to know about the tumor or the breast cancer cells in your body, they will define which stage they believe the condition to be. In most situations, doctors are able to define the stages after a few tests, but may reinforce their information with more. Over time, they will continue to monitor the situation to insure they have a full understanding of the progression of breast cancer.

Defining Treatment

Once doctors know which stage of breast cancer you are in, they can tailor your breast cancer treatments around it. This often includes several options. Whenever possible and available, they may use breast cancer surgery as their first line of defense. This will allow them to remove any types of tumors they find. In earlier stages, they may not have to remove the entire breast, either, for this to be helpful.

Doctors will nearly always combat the growth of tumors and breast cancer in general with medications. The right breast cancer drug for you will be the one that is the best at helping improving your overall health, based on the stage of your breast cancer. A wide range of treatment options are available including chemotherapy and radiation, all of which have been very helpful at improving the success rate of treatment for breast cancer.

Being educated about the level of breast cancer you have is important. Doctors will provide you with all the tools you'll need to make it through your cancer that are available, but sometimes it is not enough. The best way to avoid the worries of stage four breast cancer is to keep from getting it. Early detection is the best tool available to you. You can be a part of the successful thousands that have beaten cancer.

Cancer That Spreads

Metastatic breast cancer is a situation in which the cancer has moved from the breast tissue into the rest of the body. Because breast cancer can do this, it is highly likely that your doctor will work hard to help you avoid this happening, by giving you full body treatments for the cancer. There is usually no warning that the cancer will move. There is generally no method that shows the cancer is able to move easily or if it will not. Therefore, doctors will treat your cancer individually.

Those who are suffering from breast cancer can see metastatic situations at any time. It does not matter if you are in the early stages of breast cancer or in stage IV breast cancer. In this condition, doctors will still have treatments for breast cancer that can help you overcome the condition. Yet, they will change their scope. Many times, the goal of treating this cancer is to give you the best chance of putting the cancer into remission (non active or growing stage) while still keeping the quality of life.

Some of the treatment options for metastatic breast cancer are in the best situation if:

- The breast cancer has not spread to major organs of the body, this includes your lungs, your brain or your stomach, for example.
- The breast cancer that has spread to organs in your body has not spread to more than three organs or other parts of the body.
- The cancer will respond best if there are hormones called estrogen and progesterone hormone receptors found in the cancer cells.
- The tumor is still responding to the treatments using hormones or chemotherapy.
- And, that you have not had various types of cancer treatment or many rounds of it.

If you do not have any of these situations happening in your body, and you are concerned that treatments will not work for you, don't give up. The fact is that this type of breast cancer diagnosis is still possible to overcome. Doctors know of various ways to help treat breast cancer that has metastatic qualities to it and can often help put the cancer into remission for years to come.

The type of treatment that you'll get is dependent on various factors. For example, in some situations, breast cancer surgery can still be performed to remove any type of breast tissue that is infected, or could be infected, which would remove the cancer cells, in effect, and keep the disease from spreading. Other treatments that work well when the cancer has already spread include hormone treatments that are aggressive as well as chemotherapy treatments, especially if they were helpful in fighting the breast cancer.

The breast cancer statistics show that there are many ways that doctors can fight this condition. It does take some time to work through the process, and people do sometimes not make it through, yet, your chances of surviving and overcoming this disease are significantly higher than they were just a few years ago. Additionally, new research is readily available to help you as well.

As you consider the various options you have, consider the benefits of working with trusted doctors. If you have metastatic breast cancer, you have a new challenge, but not a life sentence. The fact is that many people are able to benefit from treatment and overcoming this disease is possible. Talk to your doctor about your individual case and learn what options in treatment are available to you. In most cases, there will be a wide range of options for doctors to select from.

Do You Know About Male Breast Cancer?

Each year, thousands of women are diagnosed with breast cancer, but there are also several hundred men that are diagnosed with male breast cancer. For those struggling with this disease, it becomes very important to consider the options you have. Perhaps the most important thing is to know that the disease is out there and that it can affect virtually any man at any time. Male breast cancer happens in only one percent of all breast cancer diagnosis each year. This amounts to about 1900 men each year. While it is a very rare disease, it is also one that needs to be closely monitored.

Learning More

Breast cancer awareness is perhaps the most important part of this disease because many men do not realize it can happen to them, and they do not realize that these conditions can affect them. Part of the study of this condition has shown that when breast cancer is detected early in the body, it can be overcome easier through the help of various methods of breast cancer treatment.

Many people believe that men do not have breasts, but in fact, they do have breast tissue. This tissue may be completely flat on your chest, in fact. In some people, the breast do develop somewhat. They may become bigger than the average man's breast, which means that they can also develop breast gland tissue, where many cancers are found. In addition to this men can experience breasts that are larger due to some medications they take, or because they have high levels of some specific types of hormones. Unfortunately, because there are not many cases of men's breast cancer, the research on this condition is limited. Yet, breast cancer research is constantly being done.

What is breast cancer? Many people are unsure about what this health scare is about. In men, breast cancer can happen because of age, with men over 60 at the highest risk. In addition, if you have a high level of estrogen, you too are at risk because cell growth is triggered by estrogen. This comes from being overweight, having liver disease or even being exposed to estrogens in the environment.

There are various types of breast cancer today, each one with its unique pattern and treatment options. Sometimes the causes of breast cancer are unknown. Other times, they can be estimated. For example, if you have a high level of exposure to radiation, this could indicate an increased risk of developing breast cancer. Family history of breast cancer can also be a reason for worry, as can exposure to products with DTT in them.

If you have been diagnosed with breast cancer, the chances of overcoming it are good. Many people find that they are able to overcome this cancer through chemotherapy, as well as other drug treatments. Doctors have a number of different types of treatment options for those suffering from breast cancer.

One of the most important tools available in the fight against breast cancer is awareness. Early detection is the key factor in saving lives, as the chances of full recovery when the cancer is detected early on is much more successful. Doctors are developing medications and treatment options that can work for nearly all cases of cancer, but getting to the doctor at the first signs of a problem are much more important. If you believe something has happened to change the breast tissue in your body, you should seek out the help of your doctor to be tested and cleared of any male breast cancer risk.

This book was written to focus on the POSITIVE side of WELLNESS so you will be a wonderful survivor (like so many women) who will keep feeling strong, healthy and optimistic throughout your cancer journey. From my own experience and research I believe that the advice and tips you'll find here will work as well for YOU, ensuring faster healing, a heightened sense of well-being and a brighter outcome.

ABOUT THE AUTHOR

Rabhu Gudapati, MD was born on July 29, 1965, and is an American neurosurgeon and an assistant professor of Medicine living in Winchester, Virginia. As an author and consultant for several health related books, he is best known as a motivational speaker who has made several appearances at a vast number of international colleges and universities. His health articles on many of the illnesses affecting persons today have been used by thousands of individuals as useful guides to return themselves to their optimum health to live healthy and normal lives.

www.ingramcontent.com/pod-product-compliance
Lightning Source LLC
Chambersburg PA
CBHW070509290526
45790CB00003B/1160